Nur Khairunnisa Nasarudin
Nor Azlina A.Rahman
Suhana Mamat

Knowledge, Attitude and Practice Regarding Dengue

AF141257

Nur Khairunnisa Nasarudin
Nor Azlina A.Rahman
Suhana Mamat

Knowledge, Attitude and Practice Regarding Dengue

A case study in Taman Temerloh Jaya, Malaysia

LAP LAMBERT Academic Publishing

Impressum / Imprint

Bibliografische Information der Deutschen Nationalbibliothek: Die Deutsche Nationalbibliothek verzeichnet diese Publikation in der Deutschen Nationalbibliografie; detaillierte bibliografische Daten sind im Internet über http://dnb.d-nb.de abrufbar.

Alle in diesem Buch genannten Marken und Produktnamen unterliegen warenzeichen-, marken- oder patentrechtlichem Schutz bzw. sind Warenzeichen oder eingetragene Warenzeichen der jeweiligen Inhaber. Die Wiedergabe von Marken, Produktnamen, Gebrauchsnamen, Handelsnamen, Warenbezeichnungen u.s.w. in diesem Werk berechtigt auch ohne besondere Kennzeichnung nicht zu der Annahme, dass solche Namen im Sinne der Warenzeichen- und Markenschutzgesetzgebung als frei zu betrachten wären und daher von jedermann benutzt werden dürften.

Bibliographic information published by the Deutsche Nationalbibliothek: The Deutsche Nationalbibliothek lists this publication in the Deutsche Nationalbibliografie; detailed bibliographic data are available in the Internet at http://dnb.d-nb.de.

Any brand names and product names mentioned in this book are subject to trademark, brand or patent protection and are trademarks or registered trademarks of their respective holders. The use of brand names, product names, common names, trade names, product descriptions etc. even without a particular marking in this works is in no way to be construed to mean that such names may be regarded as unrestricted in respect of trademark and brand protection legislation and could thus be used by anyone.

Coverbild / Cover image: www.ingimage.com

Verlag / Publisher:
LAP LAMBERT Academic Publishing
ist ein Imprint der / is a trademark of
OmniScriptum GmbH & Co. KG
Heinrich-Böcking-Str. 6-8, 66121 Saarbrücken, Deutschland / Germany
Email: info@lap-publishing.com

Herstellung: siehe letzte Seite /
Printed at: see last page
ISBN: 978-3-659-28051-1

Zugl. / Approved by: Kuantan, International Islamic University Malaysia, 2013

TABLE OF CONTENTS

Chapter 1: INTRODUCTION

Chapter 2: MATERIALS AND METHOD

Chapter 3: RESULT

Chapter 4: DISCUSSION

Chapter 5: CONCLUSION AND FUTURE WORK

LIST OF TABLES

LIST OF FIGURES

LIST OF ABBREVIATIONS

AIDS	-	Acquired Immunodeficiency Syndrome
CDC	-	Centers for Disease Control and Prevention
COMBI	-	Communication of Behavioral Impact
DALY	-	Disability-Adjusted Life Year
DENV	-	Dengue Virus
DF	-	Dengue Fever
DHF	-	Dengue Hemorrhagic Fever
DSS	-	Dengue Shock Syndrome
HIV	-	Human Immunodeficiency Virus
IQR	-	Interquartile Range
KAP	-	Knowledge, Attitude and Practice
MOH	-	Ministry of Health Malaysia
RNA	-	Ribonucleic Acid
SD	-	Standard Deviation
SPSS	-	Statistical Package for Social Science
WHO	-	World Health Organization
YLD	-	Years of Life Lived with Disability
YLL	-	Year of Life Lost

LIST OF SYMBOLS

α	-	The type I error probability
m	-	The ratio of control to experimental patients
n	-	Number of respondents/ Frequency
N	-	Total number of respondents
US$	-	Dollar of United States
%	-	Percentage
&	-	And
<	-	Less than

LIST OF APPENDICES

Chapter 1

INTRODUCTION

1.1 BACKGROUND

Dengue is a viral disease found in urban most tropical and subtropical countries in the world. A major public health problem, it is affecting 50 to 100 million world population residing in the endemic dengue area where there is constant presence of the infection. The epidemics or outbreak of dengue causes not only human suffering, but it also puts a strain on the economy and health services of a country (World Health Organization (WHO), 2012). Dengue is a vector-borne infection, transmitted principally by infective female *Aedes aegypti* and also by *Aedes albopictus* mosquito. caused by dengue viruses (DENV-1, DENV-2, DENV-3 and DENV-4) which are flaviviruses (Heymann, 2008).

In Malaysia, the first dengue case was reported in Penang in 1901 and the first case of dengue hemorrhagic fever (DHF) was reported in 1962. Since then, dengue epidemics have become more frequent throughout the country (Poovaneswari, 1993). In 2008, there were 49,335 cases with 113 deaths reported in Malaysia. It was the highest incidence in the history of dengue in this country. Consequently, the Strategic Plan of Dengue Control and Prevention had been prepared in 2009 to reduce the incidence and the burden of dengue in Malaysia (Ministry of Health Malaysia (MOH), 2009).

Temerloh District is one of the main epidemic areas of dengue in Pahang State of Malaysia. In 2007, Pahang recorded the highest dengue cases of 1,557 cases. Temerloh had recorded 156 cases in the same year and Taman Temerloh Jaya has been identified as one of the main localities of dengue in Temerloh (Asrol Awang, 2007). However, the incidence of dengue still occurs in the residential area. Currently, dengue is still the most important vector-borne disease in this country. In 2012, the incidence rate of dengue in Malaysia was 63.75 per 100,000 populations. It

1

is the highest incidence rate compared to other vector-borne diseases such as malaria and typhus (MOH, 2012).

Knowledge, Attitude and Practice (KAP) survey is a quantitative method of data collection which "quantifies and measures a phenomenon through the use of questionnaires and statistical processing of the information collected" (The KAP survey model, n.d. (p.5)). According to Kaliyaperumal (2004), the knowledge possesses by a community refers to their understanding of a health event. The attitude refers to their feeling towards the health event including any preconceived idea that they may have towards it and the practice refers to the ways they actually put their knowledge and attitude into actions.

KAP survey also discovers the factors which are often the sources of misconceptions and misunderstandings about a disease that become obstacles in promoting a health program. In addition, this survey helps to evaluate the community's behavior towards a disease and the effectiveness of health program among the community. Therefore, a KAP study was designed to collect information regarding knowledge, attitude and practice of dengue from the residents in Taman Temerloh Jaya. This study may help the public health authorities in evaluating the effectiveness of community participation in this area to control and prevent dengue. The results from this study are highly anticipated to be beneficial to the community health in this study area.

1.2 OBJECTIVE

1.2.1 General Objective

To study the knowledge, attitude and practice of dengue among the residents in Taman Temerloh Jaya, Temerloh, Pahang.

1.2.2 Specific Objectives

1. To assess the level of knowledge, attitude and practice of dengue among the study population.
2. To evaluate the relationships between knowledge, attitude and practice of dengue among the study population.
3. To determine the factors affecting knowledge, attitude and practice of dengue among the study population.

1.3 HYPOTHESIS

1. The levels of knowledge, attitude and practice of dengue among the study population are low.
2. There are significant correlations between knowledge, attitude and practice of dengue among the study population.
3. Age, race, occupation and educational level have significant associations with knowledge, attitude and practice of dengue among the study population.

1.4 LITERATURE REVIEW

1.4.1 Dengue Burden in Malaysia

Dengue infection is a major health problem and represents a large economic burden to communities and health services in a developing country such as Malaysia. Shepard, *et al.* (2013) in their review on the burden of dengue illness and its economic cost in Malaysia estimated that the total economic cost for dengue in this country is about 196 million Ringgit Malaysia (US$ 56 M) per year.

Dengue is ranked at ninth place in the top ten communicable diseases causing Disability-Adjusted Life Year (DALY) burdens in Malaysia, where this unit is used to describe the impact of a disease or injury not in just in terms of a shortened lifespan but also considering the impact on health, quantifying the resulting time spent with a reduced level of health. Dengue contributes 1.6% of all DALY burdens (8,144 DALY) in 2008 in Malaysia (Shepard, *et al*, 2013). On the other hand, according to the Ministry of Health, there were 16 deaths due to dengue fever (0.06 per 100000 population) and 118 deaths due to dengue haemorrhagic fever (0.42 per 100000 population) in Malaysia in 2010 (MOH, 2010a).

1.4.2 Manifestation of Dengue Virus Infection

The principal symptoms of dengue infection are high fever, severe headache, retro-orbital or ocular pain, myalgia or muscle pain, arthralgia or joint pain and rash. (Heymann, 2008). On the other hand, dengue hemorrhagic fever (DHF) is characterized by fever, bleeding tendencies and thrombocytopenia or low platelet counts. The capillaries can become excessively permeable causing plasma leakage which will lead to circulatory failure and shock in those patients which later can cause death. This severe condition is called dengue shock syndrome (DSS) (Centers for Disease Control and Prevention (CDC), 2014).

4

1.4.3 Transmission of Dengue Virus

Human is the most important carrier and multiplier of dengue virus, which is transmissible through the bite of a female *Aedes* mosquito after the symptoms appear in the infected person (WHO, 2014). The *Aedes* mosquito will become infected after it sucks blood with the dengue virus from a patient and can then transmit the virus to another person.

The transovarial transmission of dengue virus is an important factor to maintain the spread of the dengue virus in a population. Infected female *Aedes* mosquitoes can also transmit the virus transovarially to their offspring. Many studies confirmed that the female Aedes mosquitoes can transmit dengue virus into their offspring transovarially (Rohani, *et al*, 1997, Lee, *et al*., 1997 & Rohani, *et al*., 2007).

1.4.4 Principal Vector of Dengue

Insects that transmit diseases are called vectors. *Aedes aegypti* and *Aedes albopictus* are identified as the principal vectors of dengue in Southeast Asia (Miyagi & Toma, 2000). These species have black and white scales on their abdomens and legs (Service, 2004) that may differentiate them from other domestic mosquitoes.

Compared to *A.albopictus*, *A.aegypti* is more domestic because it breeds exclusively in artificial containers in and around human residence. It shows greater preference for indoor breeding than *A.albopictus*. Nevertheless, *A.albopictus* has also adapted to the human environment but to a lesser extent of domestication as *A.aegypti* (Miyagi & Toma, 2000; Halsted, 2008).

Both *A.aegypti* and *A.albopictus* can breed in natural and man-made artificial containers that collect rainwater and those used by human as domestic water storage as their larval habitats (Gubler & Clerk, 1996). Halsted (2008) documented that the larvae and pupae of both species can be found in clean water in many different types of artificial water containers such as tanks, jars and pots; ornamental containers such as flower holders, ant traps and shrine objects; and discarded items such as rubber tires and plastic containers.

The *Aedes* eggs were laid individually on the walls of the containers. The eggs hatch within a few minutes or up to several days after they are submerged in water. The eggs have the ability to resist desiccation for a few months. Even when the eggs were laid above the water level or without water, they are still viable and will hatch in the presence of water (Service, 2004; Halsted, 2008).

Both *A.aegypti* and *A.albopictus* have certain peak feeding periods. Female *A.aegypti* has three peaks of landing and biting activity at 7.00 am, 11.00 am, and 5.00 pm (Chadee & Martinez, 2000). Meanwhile, female *A.albopictus* bites human during daytime between 5.00 am and 7.00 pm with a main peak of activity from 3.00 pm to 7.00 pm (Kamgang, *et al.*, 2012). These studies concluded that *Aedes* mosquitoes are active during day-time and do not bite human at night.

1.4.5 Prevention and Control of Dengue

Winch, *et al.* (2002) described that there are several sets of behavior that should be promoted for preventing dengue. Elimination or control of larval habitats at the household level is one of the behaviors that have been promoted to prevent dengue. Other behaviors include self-protection from mosquito bites, early and appropriate treatment seeking, and home care for suspected cases of dengue.

These sets of behavior are also the basis for the guideline given by CDC on how to prevent dengue (CDC, 2012). Most importantly, the breeding sites of *Aedes* mosquitoes need to be eliminated. Since artificial containers are possible spots for female *Aedes* to lay eggs, it should be regularly monitored for the presence of the *Aedes* larvae. The wall of the containers should be washed with a brush to remove the eggs at least once a month. If the containers are used for water storage, they must be completely covered with a lid.

Apart from that, the application of repellants to the exposed skin is helpful to protect a person from *Aedes* mosquito bites especially during the peak biting periods. Wearing long sleeve shirts, long pants, socks and shoes during the mosquito active period is one of the good preventive measures. Window and door screens should be installed at homes to keep Aedes mosquito out. If a person in a household is infected

6

with dengue, extra precautions should be taken by other household members. For instance, the use of mosquito nets could prevent the virus transmission to other individuals in the same house.

1.4.6 Community Participation in Dengue Control and Prevention

Community participation is one of the main principles of primary health care. Among the benefits gained by community participation are people would ensure the sustainability of the health care services, contribute to support scarce resources of the health care services, control to protect their own health, and most importantly, change their poor health behavior when they explore the consequences of this behavior (Rifkin, 1996).

Gubler and Clerk (1996) described that community-based approaches provide effectiveness in controlling *Aedes* mosquitoes. It is emphasized that the effectiveness of *Aedes* control can be achieved by the community participation in reducing the presence of larval habitat of *Aedes* mosquitoes. The community should learn that they play a major role in controlling the dengue vector because they are the ones who create and tolerate the *Aedes* larval habitats in their domestic environment.

In 1999, Marina and Md. Idris (2000) conducted a study in Temerloh, Pahang to identify health behaviors that cause an increased risk of dengue by assessing the knowledge, attitude and practice regarding dengue and DHF. An association between bad health behaviors and increased risk of dengue was found in the community. The risk of getting dengue was associated with behaviors towards the use of mosquito coil and net, cleaning of water containers, larvae breeding, taking blood for testing, staying longer in hospitals for treatment, sending sick family members to hospitals and the awareness and knowledge about dengue fever.

In Puerto Rico, Winch, *et al.* (2002) studied that the community-based dengue prevention program increased the level of knowledge and awareness regarding dengue among the participants. As a result of that program, there were an increased proportion of tires protected from rain, decreased proportion of water storage

7

containers positive for mosquito larvae and increased of indoor use of aerosol insecticides by the participants.

In Malaysia, the government introduces an approach to emphasize the community participation in dengue control and prevention which is the Communication of Behavioral Impact (COMBI) approach. COMBI is utilized by mobilizing communities and resources in planning and implementing activities for the prevention and control of dengue outbreaks in dengue prone areas. This approach showed a reduced number of dengue cases in 72% of all localities where COMBI was implemented (MOH, 2010b).

1.4.7 Knowledge, Attitude and Practice Studies on Dengue

Hairi, *et al.* (2003) conducted knowledge, attitude and practice study on dengue and its vector among the selected rural communities in Kuala Kangsar, Perak. Majority of the respondents stated that the main source of information regarding dengue was television and radio. The communities had a good knowledge and good attitude towards dengue. A significant association was found between knowledge of dengue and attitude towards the vector control ($p=0.047$). The communities were also supportive to the Aedes control measures for dengue prevention. Unfortunately, there were some areas of practice which were poor among the community due to their domestic water storage. This study suggested that mass media plays an important role in spreading the information about dengue in the rural communities.

Another study was conducted by Wan Rozita, *et al.* (2006) in Kuala Lumpur among the urban communities. This study found that the communities had excellent attitude towards dengue despite of their poor knowledge and practice of dengue. There was a weak correlation between knowledge and practice of dengue ($p=0.002$). However, there was no correlation between attitude and knowledge or practice of dengue in the study population. It was concluded that good attitude does not associated with good knowledge and practice of dengue in the population. It was therefore recommended that knowledge of dengue among urban residents should be improved for better preventive practice towards dengue.

8

In Laos, a study on knowledge, attitude and practice of dengue was done by Soodsada, *et al.* (2009). The communities at 9 villages of Pakse district in Champasack Province had low level of knowledge about the vector of dengue. Their sources of information were their relatives and friends. They had good attitude towards dengue in which they believed that dengue can be treated and they were willing to visit a doctor for treatment. The villagers were quite familiar with dengue, but there was no good understanding about the prevention of dengue. Most of them kept water in a container at home but they did not change the water frequently. This study suggested that the information about dengue should be spread to the communities by the means of television and radio as well as regular visits by health personnel to the villages.

Cho, *et al.* (2011) assessed the relationship between the awareness of dengue and practice towards dengue among the semi-urban communities in Malaysia. Most of the respondents had knowledge about dengue but their practice was poor. This was due to their misconception about the vector of dengue such as they thought *Aedes* can breed in dirty water and bites human only after sunset. This study found significant associations of knowledge about dengue with age (p=0.001), educational level (p=0.001), marital status (p=0.012) and occupation (p=0.007).

Based on these previous studies, the knowledge, attitude and practice regarding dengue among the communities varied considerably. Some communities had good knowledge and attitude towards dengue but poor practice on dengue prevention. A significant association was found between knowledge and practice in some studies. There were also several socio-demographic factors which influenced the level of knowledge of dengue such as age, educational level, occupation and marital status.

Chapter 2

MATERIALS AND METHOD

2.1 STUDY DESIGN

The study design was a descriptive cross-sectional study concerning knowledge, attitude and practice of dengue among the residents of Taman Temerloh Jaya, Temerloh, Pahang.

2.2 STUDY AREA

The study was conducted in Taman Temerloh Jaya which is a semi-urban residential area located about five kilometres from the Temerloh town. It is situated about ten kilometres from the nearest hospital, Hospital Sultan Haji Ahmad Shah, Temerloh. It is one of the dengue main localities in Temerloh, Pahang during the dengue outbreak in 2007 (Asrol Awang, 2007).

2.3 STUDY POPULATION

The population in this study was the permanent residents of Taman Temerloh Jaya who had been living there for at least one year. For each house that had been approached, only one person was interviewed to represent the house. This was to avoid redundancy and inconsistency of responses.

2.4 SAMPLING METHOD

Convenience sampling was applied in this study. The subjects were recruited based on their accessibility by the researcher. This sampling method was chosen because of the limitation of time.

2.4.1 Inclusion Criteria

1. Permanent resident who had been living in for at least one year.
2. Age between 18 to 60 years old.
3. Race of Malay, Chinese or Indian.

2.4.2 Exclusion Criteria

1. Do not understand Malay or English languages.
2. Sick or mentally-ill people.

2.5 SAMPLE SIZE

A sample size of 96 was calculated using PS software version 3.0. The α level was set to be 0.05 and the standard deviation was assumed to be 7.42 based on a previous study by Wan Rozita, *et al.* (2006). The detectable difference was 5.0 and the power was 0.8. The m value was determined to be three due to the expected ratio of female to male in the population. The sample size also took into account a refusal rate of 10%. Therefore, the minimum sample size for this study was 106 subjects. The total sample size for this study was rounded off to 110 subjects.

2.6 DATA COLLECTION

The collection of data was conducted from 10th January 2013 until 30th January 2013. A face-to-face interview was done through a prepared interviewer-administered questionnaire. The interview was conducted in the local language which is Bahasa Melayu for the ease of communication between the researcher and the subjects.

2.6.1 Written Consent

Prior to the interview, explanation about the study was given and written consents were obtained from the subjects. Two copies of consent form had to be filled in by the subjects (Appendix A). One copy was given to the subject for their references and the other copy was returned to the researcher. The participation of the subjects was voluntary but they had the right to stop participating in this study at that time. They also had the right to not answering any question that makes them feel uncomfortable. Their confidentiality was assured throughout the study.

2.6.2 Questionnaire

The questionnaire was prepared and designed based on the references to the previous studies (Wan Rozita, *et al.*, 2006; Cho, *et al.*, 2011). Then, the questionnaire was reviewed by the expert in this field of study. It was prepared in English (Appendix B) but was translated into Bahasa Melayu (not included here) to be used during the interview with the subjects. The questionnaire was divided into five parts:

Part A: Socio-Demographic Information
Part B: Knowledge
Part C: Attitude
Part D: Practice
Part E: Sources of Information

The first part was regarding the socio-demographic information of the subjects. The information collected was gender, race, occupation, educational level and number of household. This information was obtained to make comparisons between the individual groups of the study population on the KAP of dengue. It was to determine the factors affecting the KAP of dengue among the study population.

The next part was on the knowledge of dengue. There were ten questions in this part concerning about the disease, the vector and the prevention of dengue. The answer choices were 'Yes', 'No' and 'I do not know'. The third part was about the attitude of the subjects towards dengue and its prevention. Eight statements were given for the subjects to agree or disagree to. The subjects could response 'Agree', 'Disagree' or 'Not sure'.

The following part asked about the preventive measures taken by the subjects to prevent and control dengue. There were seven questions and the responses were 'Everyday', 'At least once a week', 'At least once a month', 'Less than once a month' and 'Never'. The last part was about the sources of getting information about dengue. This part was to find out where the subjects got the information regarding dengue.

2.7 DATA ANALYSIS

2.7.1 Scoring System

Each response for each question in the knowledge, attitude and practice parts of the questionnaire was given a score as in Table 2.1. The score for all responses from any respondent was totaled up to get the total score for the respondent's knowledge, attitude and practice of dengue individually. The total score was used to determine the level of knowledge, attitude and practice of dengue for the individual respondents. Table 2.2 describes the level of KAP based on the total score of KAP obtained by the respondents which was modified from the Bloom's cut-off points (Nahida, 2007).

2.7.2 Statistical Analysis

The data that had been collected was analyzed by using SPSS 12.01 for Windows. Descriptive statistics (frequency, percentage, mean and standard deviation) were used to summarize and describe the socio-demographic information of the study population.

Correlation test was used to examine the relationships between knowledge and attitude, knowledge and attitude, and attitude and practice of dengue among the study population. The total score of KAP was used in this correlation test. The significant value was $p < 0.05$. The r-value determined the strength of the correlation.

Non-parametric Kruskal-Wallis test was used to compare means of total score of KAP between groups of age, race, occupation and educational level. This is because each group was not normally distributed and some of the groups had sample size less than 30. Furthermore, the population variances of some groups of analysis were not equal. p-value of less than 0.05 ($p < 0.05$) was considered as significant in this test.

Groups that showed significant result by Kruskal-Wallis test were further analyzed by post-hoc analysis using Mann-Whitney test. This statistical test compared the mean of total score of KAP between each pairs in the groups. The p-

13

value was compared to the Bonferroni concept of 0.05/ no. of pairs to find the significant pairs.

Table 2.1

Scoring system for each response of KAP

Response	Score
Knowledge	
Correct Statement	
Yes	2
No	0
I do not know	1
False Statement	
Yes	0
No	2
I do not know	1
Attitude	
Agree	2
Not sure	1
Disagree	0
Practice	
Positive practice	
Every day	4
At least once a week	3
At least once a month	2
Less than once a month	1
Never	0
Negative practice	
Every day	0
At least once a week	1
At least once a month	2
Less than once a month	3
Never	4

Table 2.2

Scoring system for level of KAP

Percentage of total score (%)	Total score of knowledge	Total score of attitude	Total score of practice	Level
80 – 100	35 – 44	13 – 16	26 – 32	Excellent
60 – 79	26 – 34	10 – 12	19 – 25	Good
40 – 59	18 – 25	6 – 9	13 – 18	Adequate
0 – 39	0 – 17	0 – 5	0 – 12	Poor

Chapter 3
RESULTS

3.1 SOCIO-DEMOGRAPHIC DISTRIBUTION

The survey questionnaire on the knowledge, attitude and practice of dengue among the residents of Taman Temerloh Jaya was completed by 110 respondents. The socio-demographic distribution of the respondents is shown in Table 3.1. Out of the 110 respondents, 80 of them were female (72.7%). The mean age of the respondents were 40 years old (SD=±12.022). Majority of the respondents were Malay (n=80, 72.7%), while the rest of them were Indian (n=18, 16.4%) and Chinese (n=12, 10.9%). Most of the respondents were housewives (n=48, 43.6%). The other non-working respondents were pensioners (n=12, 10.9%) and students (n=9, 8.2%). The working respondents were employed by the government (n=17, 15.5%), private sectors (n=14, 12.7%) and self-employed (n=10, 9.1%). More than half of the respondents had secondary educational level (n=76, 69.1%), 20 respondents had tertiary educational level (18.2%) and 14 of them only had primary educational level (12.7%). The mean number of household members among the respondents was five (SD=±2.02). About half of the respondents (n=58, 52.7%) had three to five family members who live in the same house in Taman Temerloh Jaya.

Table 3.1

Socio-demographic distribution of the respondents (N = 110)

Characteristics	Number (n)	Percentage (%)
Gender		
Male	30	27.3
Female	80	72.7
Age (years)		
18 – 25	14	12.7
26 – 35	30	27.3
36 – 45	31	28.2
46 – 55	20	18.2
56 – 60	15	13.6
Race		
Malay	80	72.7
Indian	18	16.4
Chinese	12	10.9
Occupation		
Pensioner	12	10.9
Government	17	15.5
Private	14	12.7
Self-employed	10	9.1
Housewife	48	43.6
Student	9	8.2
Educational level		
Primary	14	12.7
Secondary	76	69.1
Tertiary	20	18.2

3.2 DISTRIBUTION OF KAP LEVEL OF DENGUE

3.2.1 Knowledge of Dengue

Table 3.2 shows the distribution of knowledge level of dengue among the 110 respondents. The mean score of knowledge of dengue among the respondents were 31.25 (SD=±4.54). The knowledge score of the respondents ranged between 20 and 41. Majority of the respondents (n=72, 65.5%) had good knowledge of dengue with knowledge score between 26 and 34.

Table 3.2

Level of knowledge of dengue among respondents (N = 110)

Level (score)	Number (n)	Percentage (%)
Excellent (35 – 44)	25	22.7
Good (26 – 34)	72	65.5
Adequate (18 – 25)	13	11.8
Poor (0 – 17)	0	0

The number and percentage of the respondents for each responds regarding their knowledge of dengue were illustrated in Table 3.3. Majority of the respondents (n=105, 95.5%) knew that dengue may cause death, but some of them (n=43, 39.1%) mistakenly thought that dengue is not an infectious disease. Most of the respondents (n=94, 85.5%) correctly noticed that *Aedes* mosquito has stripes on its body. However, only 28 respondents (25.5%) knew that the vector of dengue is the female *Aedes* mosquito.

Majority of the respondents (n=106, 96.4%) knew that dengue virus is transmitted by mosquito bites. Almost half of the respondents (n=52, 47.3%) answered that water is another mode of transmission of dengue but there was 48 respondents (43.6%) who correctly responded that dengue virus cannot be transmitted by water. Half of the respondents (n=55, 50%) knew that *Aedes* mosquito does not

18

breed in dirty water and that *Aedes* mosquito can transmit the dengue virus transovarially.

More than three quarters of the respondents knew that the peak biting periods for *Aedes* mosquito are early in the morning after dawn (n=83, 75.5%) and in the evening before dusk (n=96, 87.3%). Ninety respondents (81.8%) knew that *Aedes* mosquito does not bite in the afternoon. However, there were 58 respondents who falsely thought that *Aedes* mosquito bites at night (52.7%). Majority of the respondents could correctly tell that rash (n=100, 90.9%), high fever (n=104, 94.5%) and joint pain (n=92, 83.6%) are the common symptoms of dengue fever. Nevertheless, only a few of them (n=32, 29.1%) could tell that ocular pain is another common symptom of dengue fever. Majority of the respondents (n=105, 95.5%) responded positively that the spreading of dengue virus can be overcome by removing the vector breeding sites.

Table 3.3

Knowledge of respondents regarding dengue (N =110)

Items	True n (%)	False n (%)	Don't know n (%)
1. Dengue is an infectious disease.	**63 (57.3)**	43 (39.1)	4 (3.6)
2. Dengue may lead to death.	**105 (95.5)**	3 (2.7)	2 (1.8)
3. The vector of dengue is male *Aedes* mosquito.	25 (31.8)	**28 (25.5)**	47 (42.7)
4. *Aedes* mosquito has stripes on the body.	**94 (85.5)**	4 (3.6)	12 (10.9)
5. Dengue virus can be transmitted by:			
(a) air	12 (10.9)	**82 (74.5)**	16 (14.5)
(b) water	52 (47.3)	**48 (43.6)**	10 (9.1)
(c) mosquito bite	**106 (96.4)**	0 (0)	4 (3.6)
(d) direct contact with an infected person	7 (6.4)	**91 (82.7)**	12 (10.9)

Note: The numbers highlighted in bold indicate the correct response

Table 3.3 – Continued.

	True n (%)	False n (%)	Don't know n (%)
6. *Aedes* mosquito breeds in dirty water.	50 (45.5)	**55 (50.0)**	5 (4.5)
7. Adult *Aedes* mosquito can transmit dengue virus into its eggs	**54 (49.1)**	22 (20.0)	34 (30.9)
8. The spread of dengue virus can be overcome by removing *Aedes* breeding areas.	**105 (95.5)**	1 (0.9)	4 (3.6)
9. The peak biting period of *Aedes* mosquitoes			
(a) early in the morning after dawn	**83 (75.5)**	14 (12.7)	13 (11.8)
(b) in the afternoon	4 (3.6)	**90 (81.8)**	16 (14.5)
(c) in the evening before dusk	**96 (87.3)**	6 (5.5)	8 (7.3)
(d) at night	35 (31.8)	**58 (52.7)**	17 (15.5)
10. The common symptoms of dengue fever			
(a) rash	**100 (90.9)**	2 (1.8)	8 (7.3)
(b) ocular pain	**32 (29.1)**	50 (45.5)	28 (25.5)
(c) diarrhea	50 (45.5)	**29 (26.4)**	31 (28.2)
(d) headache	85 (77.3)	**12 (10.9)**	13 (11.8)
(e) high fever	**104 (94.5)**	2 (1.8)	4 (3.6)
(f) numbness	47 (42.7)	**32 (29.1)**	31 (28.2)
(g) joint pain	**92 (83.6)**	6 (5.5)	12 (10.9)

Note: The numbers highlighted in bold indicate the correct response.

3.2.2 Attitude towards Dengue

Table 3.4 shows that majority of the respondents had an excellent attitude towards dengue (n=101, 91.8%). The mean score of attitude among the respondents was 15.21 (SD=±1.86). The minimum and maximum attitude score obtained by the respondents were 6 and 16 respectively.

Table 3.4

Level of attitude towards dengue among respondents (N = 110)

Level (score)	Number (n)	Percentage (%)
Excellent (13 – 16)	101	91.8
Good (8 – 12)	5	4.5
Adequate (6 – 9)	4	3.6
Poor (0 – 5)	0	0

The responses of the respondents on their attitudes towards dengue were demonstrated in Table 3.5. Majority of the respondents (n=106, 96.4%) agreed that their family members should work together during weekends to remove *Aedes* breeding sites. However, only 90.9% of the respondents (n =100) who actually believed that their families can help preventing dengue. Ninety nine respondents (90%) agreed that their neighbours were also responsible to prevent dengue. Many of them (n=103, 93.6%) agreed that they have the responsibility to ensure that there are no *Aedes* larvae and eggs in their housing areas. Majority of them (n=105, 95.5%) agreed that water containers must be covered properly and the inner sides of the containers should be scrubbed and clean regularly. Only 97 respondents (88.2%) agreed to open their windows and doors when fogging activities were done. Eleven respondents (10%) disagreed to give their cooperation during fogging activities. Almost all the respondents (n=108, 98.2%) had a positive attitude to bring family members who got the symptoms of dengue to see a doctor for immediate treatment.

21

Table 3.5

Attitude of respondents towards dengue (N =110)

Items	Agree n (%)	Disagree n (%)	Not sure n (%)
1. My family can help to prevent dengue.	**100(90.9)**	4 (3.6)	6 (5.5)
2. My neighbours should be responsible to prevent dengue.	**99 (90.0)**	3 (2.7)	8 (7.3)
3. Family members should spend some time during weekends to remove *Aedes* breeding sites.	**106 (96.4)**	2 (1.8)	2 (1.8)
4. It is my responsibility to make sure there are no *Aedes* eggs and/or larvae in my house area.	**103 (93.6)**	5 (4.5)	2 (1.8)
5. Water containers used for water storage must be covered properly.	**105 (95.5)**	3 (2.7)	2 (1.8)
6. The inner sides of the containers should be scrubbed and cleaned.	**105 (95.5)**	2 (1.8)	3 (2.7)
7. I shall open the doors/windows of my house during fogging activities.	**97 (88.2)**	11 (10.0)	2 (1.8)
8. If my family member has symptom of dengue fever, I will bring him/her to see a doctor for immediate treatment.	**108 (98.2)**	1 (0.9)	1 (0.9)

Note. The numbers highlighted in bold indicate the expected response.

3.2.3 Practice of Dengue

The distribution of practice level of dengue among the respondents is shown in Table 3.6. The mean score of practice level is 21.22 (SD=±6.09). The practice score ranged between 3 and 29 among the respondents. Majority of the respondents (n=49, 44.5%) had good practice on dengue prevention. Unfortunately, there were 11 respondents (10%) who had poor practice in preventing dengue.

Table 3.6

Level of practice of dengue among respondents (N =110)

Level (score)	Number (n)	Percentage (%)
Excellent (26 – 32)	31	28.2
Good (19 – 25)	49	44.5
Adequate (13 – 18)	19	17.3
Poor (0 – 12)	11	10.0

The number of respondents who used aerosol and/or liquid mosquito repellent and/or mosquito coil and/or electrical mosquito mat and/or mosquito bed net every day was 72 (65.5%). Only 42 respondents (38.2%) checked the presence of *Aedes* larvae and eggs inside and outside the house at least once a week. Majority of the respondents (n=45, 40.9%) never add larvicide into their water containers used for water storage. Most of the respondents (n=98, 89.1%) never stored water in water containers.

Majority of the respondents (n=93, 84.5%) closed their windows and doors early in the morning after dawn but 13 respondents (11.8%) never closed their windows at that period of time while the rest closed their windows and doors after dawn only at least once a week. The situation was quite the same as closing windows and doors in the evening before dusk. Majority of the respondents (n=88, 80%) closed their windows and doors during dusk but there were still some respondents (n=15, 13.6%) who never close the windows and doors during dusk. The frequency of all practices done by the respondents to prevent dengue was described in Table 3.7

Table 3.7

Practices of respondents against dengue (N =110)

Items	Every day	At least once a week	At least once a month	Less than once a month	Never
	n (%)	n (%)	n (%)	n (%)	n (%)
1. Use aerosol and/or liquid mosquito repellent and/or mosquito coil and/or electrical mosquito mat and/or mosquito bed net.	**72** **(65.5)**	32 (29.1)	3 (2.7)	2 (1.8)	1 (0.9)
2. Check for the presence of *Aedes* eggs and/or larvae inside the house.	**10** **(9.1)**	42 (38.2)	25 (22.7)	4 (3.6)	29 (26.4)
3. Check for the presence of *Aedes* eggs and/or larvae outside the house or the house compound.	**5** **(4.5)**	42 (38.2)	26 (23.6)	5 (4.5)	32 (29.1)
4. Add larvicide into the water storage containers.	**0**	25 (22.7)	22 (20.0)	18 (16.4)	45 (40.9)
5. Scrub the inner side of water storage containers.	**4** **(3.6)**	59 (53.6)	22 (20.0)	7 (6.4)	18 (16.4)
6. Store water in open containers.	4 (3.6)	2 (1.8)	1 (0.9)	5 (4.5)	**98** **(89.1)**
7. Open windows or doors					
a) early in the morning after dawn	93 (84.5)	4 (3.6)	0	0	**13** **(11.8)**
b) in the evening before dusk	88 (80.0)	7 (6.4)	0	0	**15** **(13.6)**

Note. The numbers highlighted in bold indicate the expected response.

3.3 CORRELATION BETWEEN KAP OF DENGUE

As exhibited in Table 3.8, there were significant correlations between knowledge, attitude and practice of dengue among the respondents. Knowledge of dengue had significant moderate to good correlation with attitude towards dengue ($p <0.001$; $r = +0.513$) which means that as the knowledge of dengue increases, the attitude of the respondents towards dengue also increases (Figure 3.1). There was also a significant correlation between attitude and practice of dengue ($p <0.001$; $r = +0.504$). If the person had high attitude towards dengue, the person also had excellent practice on preventing dengue (Figure 3.2). Figure 3.3 demonstrates a significant but fair correlation between knowledge and practice of dengue ($p <0.001$; $r = +0.327$).

Table 3.8

Correlation between knowledge, attitude and practice of dengue

Variables	r-value	p-value	Interpretation
Knowledge vs attitude	+0.513	<0.001	+ve moderate to good correlation
Attitude vs practice	+0.504	<0.001	+ve moderate to good correlation
Knowledge vs practice	+0.327	<0.001	Fair positive correlation

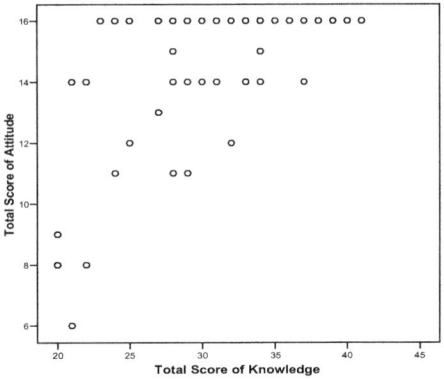

Figure 3.1

Correlation between knowledge and attitude of dengue

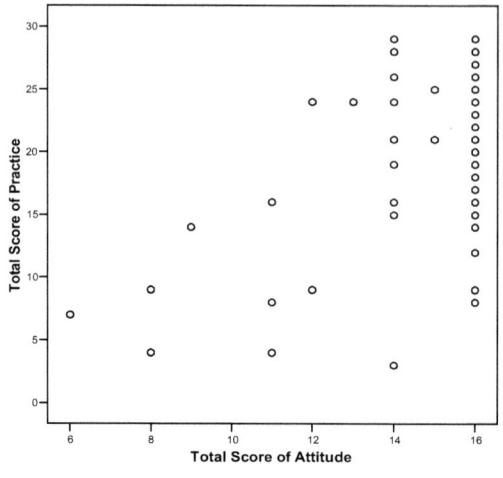

Figure 3.2

Correlation between attitude and practice of dengue

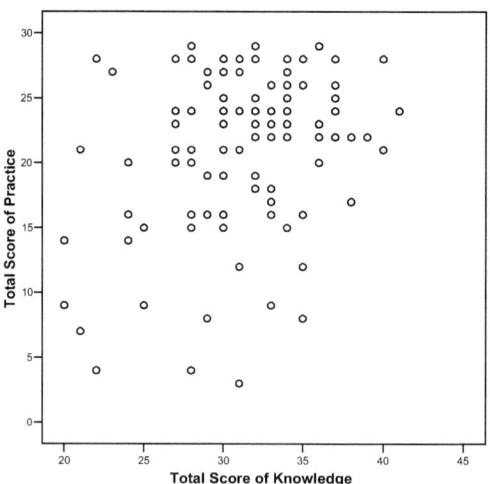

Figure 3.3

Correlation between knowledge and practice of dengue

3.4 ASSOCIATION OF SOCIO-DEMOGRAPHIC FACTORS WITH KAP OF DENGUE

3.4.1 Comparing Knowledge of Dengue between Different Groups of Age, Race, Occupation and Educational Level

Based on Table 3.9, it is shown that only age (p =0.005) and educational level (p =0.034) had significant differences of the mean score of knowledge of dengue.

Table 3.9

Comparison of knowledge of dengue between different groups of age, race, occupation and educational level

Variables	n	Median (IQR)	Test statistics value (df)	p-value*
Age (years)				
18 – 25	14	30 (7)	14.993 (4)	**0.005**
26 – 35	30	29 (5)		
36 – 45	31	33 (4)		
46 – 55	20	34 (5)		
56 – 60	15	32 (6)		
Race				
Malay	80	32.5 (4)	5.639 (2)	0.060
Indian	18	29.5 (12)		
Chinese	12	28.5 (9)		
Occupation				
Housewife	48	32.5 (7)	4.313 (5)	0.505
Government	17	33 (7)		
Private	14	31.5 (8)		
Pensioner	12	32 (6)		
Self-employed	10	30.5 (7)		
Student	9	30 (8)		

Note. *Kruskal-wallis test

Table 3.9 : continued

Variables	n	Median (IQR)	Test statistics value (df)	*p*-value*
Educational level				
Primary	15	28 (11)	6.74 (2)	**0.034**
Secondary	75	32 (5)		
Tertiary	20	32.5 (4)		

Note. *Kruskal-wallis test

Table 3.10 shows that there were significant differences in two pairs of age group which are between the pairs of 26 – 35 and 36 – 45 (p <0.001) and 26 – 35 and 46 – 55 (p =0.004). Post-hoc analysis between pairs of educational level for differences in knowledge of dengue is shown in Table 3.11. There was a significant difference found between primary level and secondary level of education (p =0.017) and between primary level and tertiary level of education (p =0.019).

Table 3.10

Post-hoc analysis for knowledge of dengue between age groups

Pairs	*p*-value*
18 – 25 and 26 – 35	0.526
18 – 25 and 36 – 45	0.063
18 – 25 and 46 – 55	0.118
18 – 25 and 56 – 60	0.283
26 – 35 and 36 – 45	**<0.001**
26 – 35 and 46 – 55	**0.004**
26 – 35 and 56 – 60	0.073
36 – 45 and 46 – 55	0.876
36 – 45 and 56 – 60	0.430
46 – 55 and 56 – 60	0.432

Note. * Mann-Whitney test

Table 3.11

Post-hoc analysis for knowledge of dengue between educational levels

Pairs	p-value*
Primary – Secondary	**0.017**
Primary – Tertiary	**0.019**
Secondary – Tertiary	0.554

Note. * Mann-Whitney test

3.4.2 Comparing Attitude of Dengue between Different Groups of Age, Race, Occupation and Educational Level

Table 3.12 exhibits that race (p <0.001) and educational level (p =0.014) had significant association with attitude of dengue among the study population.

Table 3.12

Comparison of attitude of dengue between different groups of age, race, occupation and educational level

Variables	n	Median (IQR)	Test statistics value (df)	p-value*
Age (years)				
18 – 25	14	16 (2)	5.532 (4)	0.237
26 – 35	30	16 (1)		
36 – 45	31	16 (0)		
46 – 55	20	16 (0)		
56 – 60	15	16 (4)		
Race				
Malay	80	16 (0)	24.72 (2)	**<0.001**
Indian	18	16 (1)		
Chinese	12	13.5 (5)		

Note. * Kruskal-Wallis test

29

Table 3.12 : continued

Variables	n	Median (IQR)	Test statistics value (df)	p-value*
Occupation				
Housewife	48	16 (0)	11.137 (5)	0.049
Government	17	16 (0)		
Private	14	16 (0)		
Pensioner	12	16 (3)		
Self-employed	10	16 (0)		
Student	9	14 (2)		
Educational level				
Primary	15	16 (5)	8.541 (2)	**0.014**
Secondary	75	16 (0)		
Tertiary	20	16 (0)		

Note. * Kruskal-Wallis test

There was a significant difference between Malay and Chinese ($p < 0.001$) in terms of their attitude towards dengue (Table 3.13). It is shown in Table 3.14 that the residents who had only primary education had significantly different level of attitude towards dengue compared to those residents who had secondary level ($p = 0.008$) and tertiary level ($p = 0.017$) of education.

Table 3.13

Post-hoc analysis for attitude of dengue between races

Pairs	p-value*
Malay – Indian	0.314
Malay – Chinese	**<0.001**
Indian – Chinese	0.024

Note. * Mann-Whitney test

Table 3.14

Post-hoc analysis for attitude of dengue between educational levels

Pairs	p-value*
Primary – Secondary	**0.008**
Primary – Tertiary	**0.017**
Secondary – Tertiary	0.525

Note. * Mann-Whitney test

3.4.3 Comparing Practice of Dengue between Different Groups of Age, Race, Occupation and Educational Level

Based on Table 3.15, it is shown that race (p <0.001) and educational level (p =0.004) had significant associations with the practice of dengue among the study population.

Table 3.15

Comparison of practice of dengue between different groups of age, race, occupation and educational level

Variables	n	Median (IQR)	Test statistics value (df)	p-value*
Age (years)				
18 – 25	14	22.5 (6)	2.148 (4)	0.709
26 – 35	30	24 (8)		
36 – 45	31	22 (10)		
46 – 55	20	24 (9)		
56 – 60	15	22 (8)		
Race				
Malay	80	24 (6)	22.622 (2)	**<0.001**
Indian	18	16.5 (12)		
Chinese	12	16 (16)		

Note. * Kruskal-Wallis test

Table 3.15 : continued

Occupation				
Housewife	48	22.5 (10)	2.494 (5)	0.777
Government	17	22 (5)		
Private	14	24 (11)		
Pensioner	12	23 (10)		
Self-employed	10	26 (11)		
Student	9	21 (7)		
Educational level				
Primary	15	16 (15)	11.149 (2)	**0.004**
Secondary	75	22 (8)		
Tertiary	20	25.5 (5)		

Note. * Kruskal-Wallis test

Table 3.16 shows that there were significant differences between races of Malay and Indian (p =0.002) and Malay and Chinese (p <0.001) in terms of practice of dengue among the respondents. There were also significant differences in the practice of dengue between primary and tertiary educational levels (p =0.004) and between secondary and tertiary educational levels (p =0.013) as shown in Table 3.17. There was no difference between the practice of primary and secondary groups of the residents in this study.

Table 3.16

Post-hoc analysis for practice of dengue between races

Pairs	p-value*
Malay – Indian	**0.002**
Malay – Chinese	**<0.001**
Indian – Chinese	0.243

Note. * Mann-Whitney test

32

Table 3.17

Post-hoc analysis for practice of dengue between educational levels

Pairs	p-value*
Primary – Secondary	0.045
Primary – Tertiary	**0.004**
Secondary – Tertiary	**0.013**

Note. * Mann-Whitney test

3.5 SOURCES OF INFORMATION

Figure 3.4 shows the distribution of the respondents by different sources of information about dengue. The respondents got the information regarding dengue from television (TV) or radio (n =104, 96.3%), followed by newspaper or magazine (n =99, 90.0%), health staff (n =90, 81.8%), poster (n =71, 64.5%), family and friends (n =61, 55.5%), neighbours (n =59, 53.6%), internet (n =40, 36.4%) and brochure (n =40, 36.4%).

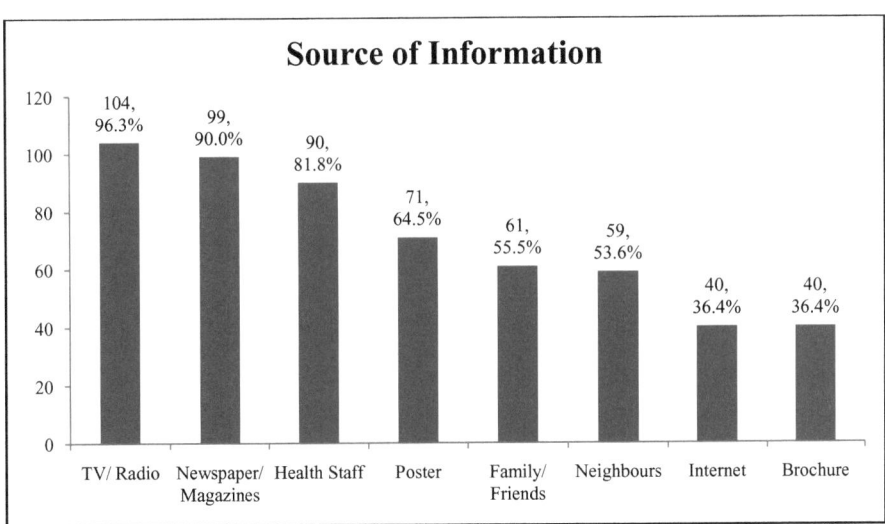

Figure 3.4

Sources of information about dengue (N =110)

33

Chapter 4

DISCUSSION

4.1 Socio-Demographic Characteristics

Majority of the respondents were female because it was mostly women who were available during the time of interview. It was difficult to interview a male respondent because most of them were working. Therefore, they were not at home during the interview. For some who were at home, they asked their wives to give responses as they claimed women know better about their houses and family health.

Mostly, the residents were those who work and have a family in the age range between 26 and 55 years old while some respondents were younger in the age range from 18 to 25 years old. They were most probably students who were living together with their parents. The rest of the respondents were older people in the age range of a retiree which is between 56 to 60 years old. Majority of the respondents were Malay which represents majority of the residents in Taman Temerloh Jaya. Only 18 Indian respondents and 12 Chinese respondents were interviewed because it was quite difficult to get their consent and the refusal rate was higher among Chinese residents.

Furthermore, it was mostly housewives who had been interviewed about the KAP of dengue because they were the ones who were available at their houses. They were the ones who responsible to look after their family and houses every day. Other females and majority of males were working with the government or private sectors, or they were having their own business. The rest of them were students and pensioners.

Most of the residents had secondary level of education. It is common among the residents as most of them were older people who did not have the same chance to further study at tertiary level of education as the younger generation. About 20% of the respondents had tertiary level of education. Those with higher educational level were expected to have better level of knowledge, attitude and practice regarding dengue. Minority of the respondents had only primary level of education.

4.2 Knowledge, Attitude and Practice Level of Dengue

The results from this study showed that knowledge of the respondents about dengue was good. This might be because the respondents got much information about dengue from various sources including television and radio. Television and radio was the most popular source of information regarding dengue among the study population. This result was similar to the result of the study by Hairi, *et al*. (2003). They found that the communities in rural areas had good knowledge about dengue and they got information mostly from television and radio.

According to the responses of the subjects in the questionnaire, the areas where majority of the respondents could answer correctly were the impact of severe dengue infection, the mode of transmission of the virus, the peak biting period of *Aedes* mosquitoes, the common symptoms of dengue fever and the method of preventing the spread of dengue. Meanwhile, some of the respondents showed lack of knowledge regarding the vector which is the *Aedes* mosquitoes.

Most of the respondents did not know which sex of Aedes mosquito bites human and transmits the dengue virus. Some of them thought that male Aedes mosquitoes were the ones that spread the disease. Most of them also did not know that female Aedes mosquitoes can transmit the virus into their offspring. It was important to know about the transovarial transmission of dengue virus because one of the ways to prevent the disease is by removing or eliminating the *Aedes* breeding sites around houses. By this way, the *Aedes* eggs or larvae which contain the virus can be prevented from growing into an adult mosquito and infecting human.

Despite that most of them knew that *Aedes* mosquito is the vector of dengue, some of them mistakenly thought that dengue virus can also be transmitted by water. They had misconception that dengue able to spread through water because they were informed to remove stagnant water as a method of prevention. Apparently, there was some confusion among some of the respondents about the transmission of the disease. These findings showed that some of the respondents only followed what they were advised to do to prevent dengue without understanding the significance of this practice. For example, removing any stagnant water does not mean that the water can cause dengue but the water may contain eggs and larvae of *Aedes* which had been infected with the virus.

Nevertheless, majority of the respondents could correctly answered that dengue virus is transmitted by mosquito bites. Surprisingly, a large group of the respondents responded falsely that dengue is not an infectious disease. This situation might be due to their misunderstanding of the term 'infectious disease' in the question given to them. The respondents may falsely understand that 'infectious disease' means 'contagious disease'. This is because both terms are translated into the same term as *'penyakit berjangkit'* in Bahasa Melayu. This term was used during the interview but it actually meant 'infectious disease'. In the future, simpler term should be used to avoid misconception among the residents who had low scientific knowledge.

The respondents in this study were found to have excellent attitude towards preventing dengue. This result was supported by previous study conducted by Wan Rozita, *et al.* (2006) who found that the urban community in Kuala Lumpur also had good attitude towards dengue. For instance, the community was cooperative during fogging activities that were done in their areas. The respondents in Taman Temerloh Jaya were agreed to bring their family members who have symptoms of dengue to the hospital immediately for treatment. This finding was similar to the attitude of the villagers in Pakse, Laos where majority of them will go to see a doctor if they are sick and have any symptoms of dengue infection (Soodsada, *et al.*, 2009).

It was found in this study that the residents had good practice towards dengue. This contrasted previous KAP studies on dengue done in semi-urban and urban areas in Malaysia where majority of the respondents had poor practice of preventing dengue (Wan Rozita, *et al.*, 2006; Cho, *et al.*, 2011). The good practice among the residents of Taman Temerloh Jaya may be due to their awareness on dengue had developed after the dengue outbreak in 2007.

Based on the analysis of the responses, the respondents seemed to focus on getting rid of *Aedes* adult mosquitoes rather than the eggs and larvae. For example, many of them never use larvicides to kill *Aedes* eggs and larvae but most of them frequently used mosquito repellents or mosquito coils or mat in order to get rid the adult mosquitoes. In addition, majority of them did not frequently check for the presence of *Aedes* eggs and larvae. Only a few of them scrub the inner wall of their water storage every week.

One of the reasons why the respondents chose to combat with the adult mosquito preferably might be due to the availability of mosquito repellents compared to larvicides in the market. Commonly, the respondents only got the larvicides from the public health staff that checked for the presence of *Aedes* larvae and eggs in their housing areas. They did not take the initiative to buy and put the larvicides into their water containers by their own. Furthermore, there were not many of the residents who stored water in containers because they did not want to be fined if they were found to have *Aedes* larvae and eggs in those containers. These reasons were based on the comments from the residents during the interview session. It may not be true so further investigations should be done in the future.

4.3 Correlation between KAP of Dengue

It was found that the knowledge, attitude and practice of dengue among the study population were at a good level. Interestingly there were positive correlations between KAP of dengue. Based on the comparison between knowledge to the attitude of dengue in the study population, it was found that higher knowledge contributed to the better attitude. This result implied that someone who knew more about dengue had better attitude towards dengue. On the other hand, someone who had lack of knowledge about dengue had lower attitude in preventing dengue.

Next, there were correlation between attitude and practice of dengue in this study population. This explained that those who had better attitude would also have better practice towards dengue. For example, majority of the respondents who agreed that they have responsibility to check for the presence of Aedes eggs and larvae in their house areas would do so. However, those who did not care about dengue would do nothing to prevent dengue.

Positive correlation was also found between knowledge and practice of dengue among the respondents. However, they were weakly correlated to each other. It was consistent with the result from the study by Wan Rozita, *et al.* (2006) which also found a weak correlation between knowledge and practice of dengue among the study population. Better knowledge also leads to better practice in some ways. For instance, someone who knew that *Aedes* mosquito only bites during after dawn and before dusk would close their windows and doors during that time. But, for someone who thought that *Aedes* mosquito only active at night would let their windows and doors open in the morning after dawn.

4.4 Factors Associating with KAP of Dengue

Based on the result of this study, there were some socio-demographic factors which were associated with the knowledge, attitude and practice of dengue among the study population. All factors that were tested in this study had significant association with knowledge, attitude and dengue except occupation, which did not show any association with knowledge, attitude or practice of dengue.

Age was found to be the determinant of knowledge about dengue. Due to the small sample size and different sample size between each age group, only two age groups were found significantly different in terms of knowledge of dengue. Young adults aged between 26 to 35 years old had different level of knowledge compared to the middle-aged adults between 36 to 55 years old. The middle-aged group was found to have better knowledge compared to the young adults. This result was inconsistent with the founding by Cho, *et al.* (2011) whereby they found that older people in the study area tends to have poor knowledge compared to younger people.

The second important factor which affects the knowledge, attitude and practice of dengue is educational level. Higher education level results in better knowledge, attitude and practice of dengue in this study population. It was found from the statistical analysis that in terms of knowledge and attitude, there were significant differences between the primary educational level group with secondary and tertiary educational groups. People with primary education had lower knowledge and attitude towards dengue. This result was supported by the positive correlation found between knowledge and attitude of dengue.

However, people with secondary educational level had no difference in the practice towards dengue with people who had primary education. But, those who had secondary education had a significant difference with those who had tertiary education. The tertiary education people showed better practice compared to secondary and primary education people. This was related to the weak correlation between knowledge and practice of dengue in this study population. Though the secondary education group had better knowledge and attitude regarding dengue, they did not necessarily have good practice of dengue.

Another factor that was tested in this study is race. There was no significant difference in knowledge of dengue among the races of Malay, Indian and Chinese in this residential area. However, significant associations were found between race and the attitude as well as practice towards dengue. Malays had better attitude towards dengue compared to Chinese. Due to small sample size in Indian and Chinese groups, no difference was found between the two groups in terms of their attitude. Regarding the practice of dengue, Malays were found to have better practice compared to Indian and Chinese in this population.

4.5 Limitations of the Study

The results of this study could not be generalized to the whole population in Temerloh, Pahang because it involved a small sample size. Furthermore, convenience sampling was applied instead of random sampling due to limitation of time and cost. Therefore, this study was prone to selection bias where the person with higher or lower KAP might be missed from this study. As a result, the determination of the level of KAP about dengue in this study population may not be accurate. It may overestimate the actual level of KAP in the study population. Nonetheless, this study can be a pilot study to determine the level of knowledge, attitude and practice of dengue among the semi-urban community in Temerloh, Pahang.

Chapter 5
CONCLUSION AND FUTURE WORK

5.1 CONCLUSION

This is a pilot study done to access the knowledge, attitude and practice of dengue among the residents in Taman Temerloh Jaya, Temerloh, Pahang. It was found that the level of knowledge, attitude and practice of dengue among the selected respondents was good. Good behavior towards dengue had been developed by the residents from the information they got about dengue and its prevention. However, there was some misunderstanding about the transmission of dengue virus. The attitude of the study population towards dengue was categorized as excellent but it was not translated well into practice. The study population paid more attention on controlling the adult mosquito than the *Aedes* eggs and larvae. Positive correlations were established between knowledge, attitude and practice of dengue of the study population. Educational level, race and age were the factors that associated with knowledge, attitude and practice of dengue but occupation failed to show any association with knowledge, attitude or practice of dengue.

The results of this study suggested that the residents in a dengue epidemic area may develop good knowledge, attitude and practice of dengue due to previous outbreak. However, there were some aspects regarding the control of dengue vector that need to be scaled up to improve the knowledge and behavior of the residents towards prevention of dengue. This could be achieved by utilizing mass media in spreading the information of dengue control and prevention to the residents.

5.2 FUTURE WORK

As for related and similar study to be done in the future, a larger sample size is needed in order to obtain more accurate results and lower the standard deviation. Furthermore, larger sample size could represent the true population in the study area. The questionnaire should be more comprehensive and include questions that will give data about the vector, the transmission of virus, the disease and the method of control and prevention that was adapted by the respondents in each part of knowledge, attitude and practice.

Next, more studies on the knowledge, attitude and practice of dengue should be conducted in other dengue epidemics area to compare the results of the studies. A comparison study with other residential area which is free from dengue epidemic should also be conducted to see the differences of KAP among the residents. Studies that concentrate on the factors that affect the KAP of dengue could also be done with a larger and equal sample size between each group of the factor such as age, gender, occupation, educational level, marital status and race to get more reliable results.

REFERENCES

Asrol Awang. (2007). Kuantan lubuk denggi. *Harian Metro Online*. Retrieved from
http://hkulim.moh.gov.my/modules/news/makepdf.php?storyid=88

Centers for Disease Control and Prevention. (2012, May 4). *Prevention*. Retrieved
from Dengue Homepage: http://www.cdc.gov/Dengue/prevention/index.html

Centers for Disease Control and Prevention. (2014, August 5). *Clinical Descriptions
for Case Definitions*. Retrieved from Dengue Homepage:
http://www.cdc.gov/dengue/clinicalLab/caseDef.html

Chadee, D. D., & Martinez, R. (2000). Landing periodicity of Aedes aegypti with
implications for dengue transmissionin Trinidad, West Indies. *Journal of
Vector Ecology*, 158-162.

Cho, N., Wong, Y. R., Chan, Y. M., Koh, P. F., Chua, Q., Choo, N. N., & Clarice, W.
S. (2011). Awareness of Dengue and Practice of Dengue Control Among the
Semi-Urban Community: A Cross Sectional Survey. *Journal of Community
Health, 36*(6), 1044-1049.

Gubler, D. J., & Clerk, G. G. (1996). Community involvement in the control of
Aedes aegypti. *Acta Tropica, 61*, 169-179.

Hairi, F., Ong, H. S., Suhaimi, A., Tsung, T. W., Anis Ahmad, M. A., Sundaraj, C., &
Soe, M. M. (2003). A Knowledge, Attitude and Practices (KAP) Study on
Dengue among Selected Rural Communities in the Kuala Kangsar District.
Asia-Pacific Journal of Public Health, 15(1), 37-43.

Halstead, S. B. (2008). Epidemiology. In S. B. Halstead (Ed.), *Dengue* (pp. 75-122).
London: Imperial College Press.

Heymann, D. L. (Ed) (2008). *Control of Communicable Diseases Manual (4th Ed.)*.
Washington : American Public Health Association.

Kaliyaperumal, K. (2004). Guideline for Conducting a Knowledge,Attitude and
Practice (KAP) study. *AECS Illumination*, 4(1), pp. 7-9.

Kamgang, B., Nchoutpouen, E., Simard, F., & Paupy, C. (2012). Notes on the blood-feeding behavior of Aedes albopictus (Diptera: Culicidae) in Cameroon. *Parasites and Vectors, 5*(57), pp. 1-4.

Lee, H. L., Mustafakamal, I., & Rohani, A. (1997). Does transovarian transmission of dengue virus occur in Malaysian Aedes Aegypti and Aedes Albopictus? *Southeast Asean Journal Tropical Medicine Public Health, 28*, 230-232.

Marina, B., & Md. Idris, M. N., (2000). Health Behavior and its Relationship with The Risk of Getting Dengue Fever at the District of Temerloh Pahang Darul Makmur:A Case Control Study, 1999. Retrieved from: *journalarticle.ukm.my/4580/1/Vol12(1)-Kasemani.pdf*

Ministry of Health Malaysia. (2009). *Pelan Strategi Kawalan dan Pencegahan Denggi.* pp.1-18, Putrajaya : Ministry of Health.

Ministry of Health Malaysia. (2010a). *Country Health Plan: 10th Malaysian Plan (2011-2015).* p.14, Putrajaya : Ministry of Health.

Ministry of Health Malaysia. (2010b). *Health Indicators 2010.*Putrajaya : Ministry of Health.

Ministry of Health Malaysia. (2012). *Health Facts 2012.* p. 5, Putrajaya : Ministry of Health.

Miyagi, I., & Toma, T. (2000). The Mosquitoes of Southeast Asia. In F. Ng, & H. S. Yong (Eds.), *Mosquitoes and mosquito-borne disease* (p. 10). Kuala Lumpur: Academy of Sciences Malaysia.

Nahida, A. (2007). Knowledge, Attitude and Practice of Dengue Fever Prevention among the people in Male', Maldives. Master Thesis. Chulalongkorn University.

Poovaneswari, S. (1993). Dengue Situation in Malaysia. *Malaysian Journal of Pathology, 15*(1), 3-7.

Rifkin, S. B., (1996). Paradigms Lost: Toward a New Understanding of Community Participation in Health Programmes. *Acta Tropica,* 61, 79-92.

Rohani, A., Asmaliza, S. I., Zainah, S., Ravindran, T., & Lee, H. L. (1997). Detection of dengue virus from field Aedes aegypti and Aedes albopictus adults and larvae. *Southeast Asian Journal Tropical Medicine Public Health, 28*, 138-142.

Rohani, A., Zamree, I., Lee, H. L., Mustafakamal, I., Norjaiza, M. J., & Kamilan, D. (2007). Detection of transovarial dengue virus in field-caught Aedes aegypti and Aedes albopictus mosquitoes using C6/36 cell culture and reverse transcriptase-polymerase chain reaction (RT-PCR) techniques. *Dengue Bulletin, 41*, 47-56.

Service, M. W. (2004). *Medical Entomology for Students* (Vol. III). Cambridge University Press.

Shepard, D. S., Lees, R., Ng, C. W., Undurraga, E. A., Lara, H., & Lum, L. (2013, March 18th). *Burden of Dengue in Malaysia: Report from a Collaboration between Universities and the Ministry of Health of Malaysia.* Retrieved from http://www.google.com.my/url?sa=t&rct=j&q=&esrc=s&source=web&cd=3& ved=0CC8QFjAC&url=http%3A%2F%2Fpeople.brandeis.edu%2F~shepard% 2FReport_dengue_in_Malaysia_v50.pdf&ei=bfzeU-_7Oc-fugSfjYKADA&usg =AFQjCNGi5djlCe3kmj2DluN-BevCluNCqw&bvm=bv.72197243,d.c2E

Soodsada, N., Yoshitoku, Y., Satoshi, M., Keo, S., & Junichi, S. (2009). Knowledge, Attitude and Practice Regarding Dengue among People in Pakse, Laos. *Nagoya Journal Medicine Science, 71*, 29-37.

The KAP survey model (n.d). Retrieved from: http://www.medecinsdumonde.org/ content/download/1772/13753/file/6c27001736f069d23fab6b06b30ee3a1.pdf

Wan Rozita, W. M., Yap, B. W., Veronica, S., Muhammad, A. K., Lim, K. H., & Sumarni, M. G. (2006). Knowledge, Attitude and Practice (KAP) Survey on Dengue Fever in an Urban Malay Residential Area in Kuala Lumpur. *Malaysian Journal of Public Health Medicine, 6*(2), 62-67.

Winch, P. J., Leontsini, E., Rigau-Perez, J. G., Clark, G. G., & Gubler, D. J. (2002). Community-Based Dengue Prevention Programmes in Puerto Rico: Impact of Knowledge, Behavior and Residential Mosquito Infestation. *American Journal of Tropical Medicine and Hygiene*, 67(4), 363-370.

World Health Organization (2012). *Global Strategy For Dengue Prevention And Control.* Geneva : WHO Press.

World Health Organization (2014, August 5). *Dengue Control.* Retrieved from the World Health Organization website: http://www.who.int/denguecontrol/human/en/

APPENDIX A: CONSENT FORM

CONSENT FORM

Research Title:	**Knowledge, Attitude and Practice of Dengue among Residents in Taman Temerloh Jaya, Temerloh.**
Researcher:	Nur Khairunnisa Nasarudin
	Department of Biomedical Science, IIUM.
Supervisor:	Dr. Suhana Mamat
	Department of Biomedical Science, IIUM.
Co-supervisor:	Dr. Nor Azlina A Rahman
	Department of Biomedical Science, IIUM.

This is to state that I agree to participate in this research study. I have been informed that:

- The purpose of this study is to evaluate the level of knowledge, attitude and practice of dengue among the residents of Taman Temerloh Jaya, Temerloh.
- I must be at least 18 years of age and had been living in Taman Temerloh Jaya for at least one year to participate in this study.
- I will be interviewed to answer a few questions to complete the questionnaire.
- The participation in this study will not exceed 30 minutes.
- My participation is voluntary. I have the right to withdraw my consent and stop participating at any time. I may choose not to answer questions that make me feel uncomfortable.
- My participation is confidential. My identity will not be revealed in the study result.
- The data from this study may be published. However, it will be presented in group form.

I have read and understand all the information provided in this form and freely consent to participate in this study.

Name: _____

IC No: _____

Contact No: _____

Signature: _____   Date: _____

Ref. No: _____

KNOWLEDGE, ATTITUDE & PRACTICE OF DENGUE AMONG RESIDENTS IN TAMAN TEMERLOH JAYA, TEMERLOH

PART A: SOCIO-DEMOGRAPHIC INFORMATION

1. Gender:	Male		Female			
2. Age:						
3. Race:	Malay		Indian		Chinese	
4. Occupation:	Medical Staff		Teacher		Businessman	
	Housewife		Others (please state)			
5. Educational level:	Primary education		Secondary education		Tertiary education	
6. No. of household members:						

PART B: KNOWLEDGE

No	Question	True	False	Do not know
1.	Dengue is an infectious disease.			
2.	Dengue may lead to death.			
3.	The vector of dengue is male *Aedes* mosquito.			
4.	*Aedes* mosquito has stripes on the body.			
5.	Dengue virus can be transmitted by:			
	(a) air			
	(b) water			
	(c) mosquito bite			
	(d) direct contact with an infected person			
6.	*Aedes* mosquito breeds in dirty water.			
7.	Adult *Aedes* mosquito can transmit dengue virus into its eggs.			
8.	The peak biting period of *Aedes* mosquitoes is:			
	(a) early in the morning after dawn			
	(b) in the afternoon			
	(c) in the evening before dusk			
	(d) at night			
9.	The common symptoms of dengue fever are:			
	(a) rash			
	(b) eye pain			
	(c) diarrhea			
	(d) headache			
	(e) high fever			
	(f) numbness			
	(g) joint pain			
10.	The spread of dengue virus can be overcome by removing *Aedes* breeding areas.			

PART C: ATTITUDE

No.	Statement	Agree	Disagree	Not sure
1.	My family can help to prevent dengue.			
2.	My neighbours should have the responsibility to prevent dengue.			
3.	Family members should spend some time during the weekends to remove *Aedes* breeding sites.			
4.	It is my responsibility to make sure that there is no *Aedes* egg and/or larva in my house area.			
5.	Water containers for water storage must be covered properly.			
6.	The inner sides of the containers used for water storage should be scrubbed and cleaned.			
7.	I shall open the doors/windows of my house during fogging.			
8.	If my family member has symptoms of dengue fever, I will bring him/her to see a doctor for immediate treatment.			

PART D: PRACTICE

No.	Statement	Every day	At least once a week	At least once a month	Less than once a month	Never
1.	Use aerosol and/or liquid mosquito repellent and/or mosquito coil and/or electrical mosquito mat and/or mosquito bed net.					
2.	Check for the presence of *Aedes* eggs and/or larvae inside the house.					
3.	Check for the presence of *Aedes* eggs and/or larvae outside the house or the house compound.					
4.	Add larvicides into the water storage containers.					
5.	Scrub the inner side of water storage containers.					
6.	Store water in open containers.					
	Open windows or doors					
7.	(a) early in the morning after dawn					
	(b) in the evening before dusk					

PART E: SOURCES OF INFORMATION ON DENGUE

How do you get information regarding dengue?

(More than one (1) answer can be chosen)

TV / radio	
Poster / billboard	
Internet (websites)	
Newspaper / magazines	
Brochure / pamphlet	
Family / friends	
Neighbours	
Health staff	
Others. Specify :	

Thank you very much for your participation. May God bless you!

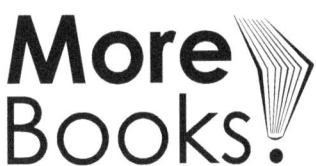
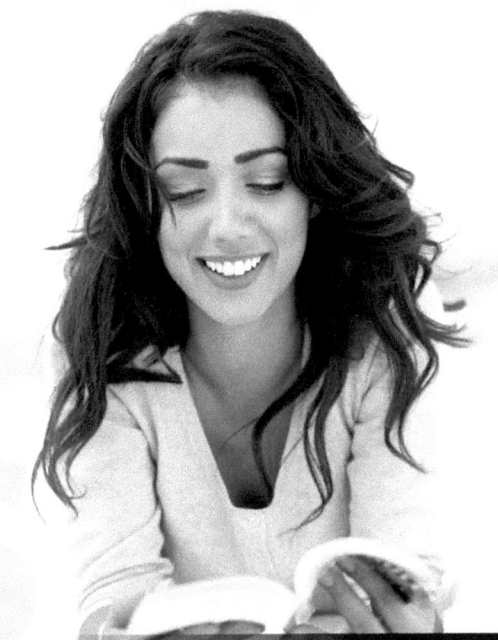

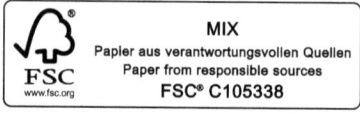